INSIDE COVID

My Personal Journey

JEROME A. CARTER

Table of Contents

Introduction

I want to establish a theme at the beginning so there is no misunderstanding throughout this journey. I am writing this journey from a P.O.P.E perspective. What is a P.O.P.E. perspective? It is (P) ersonally (O) bserved (P) ersonally (E) xperienced. This perspective is from the inside out and can't be experienced except by the person going through the process. This experience is not from a book or an article written by an unknown person. Some people may read a book or read an article and think they know about a particular subject. When in reality they have never experienced it. They can only go by what they have read.

Well, this is not that type of book. This is my journey, how I felt and how others felt and responded to the situation. Also, know that everything you will read in this book is factual. These events are part of my journey. This book is not a formal or clinical explanation of Covid. However, there may be clinical terms and descriptions to describe an event.

Also, there needs to be a foundation established when I talk about Covid. Covid has many different strains and those strains affect people in different ways. Some people may just have a common cold reaction, while others may have to be hospitalized. Then there are the ones who need to have a medically induced coma to deal with the virus. One of the things that make this virus difficult is that it has different reactions to different people. These variations cause confusion and disbelief especially when a person gets deathly ill or dies.

Most people don't know there are many different types of Covid. So, with that said, my journey might not be special or one of a kind but it must be told. Some people don't believe the virus is real and how it is affecting families and friends. The message coming out is cloudy and muddy because of those disagreements. What I find amazing is no one thinks the common flu virus is a hoax or not real. On the other hand, covid is fifty-fifty if it is real. That, in itself, is a problem. But I digress. Be it good or be it bad, here is my journey.

CHAPTER ONE
Not Me I'm Good

Like most men who are 45 years old and work out weekly, I felt strong. Yes, covid was making its rounds and it was not going to affect me. I trained myself to overcome physical and mental obstacles. In the past, I have gotten sick and had to get outpatient treatment for breathing issues related to allergies. I'm familiar with albuterol, nebulizers, and Zyrtec D. I also know the importance of the three fluids in your body that need constant moving to prevent sickness. Those three fluids are blood, bile, and mucus.

I was drinking kombucha and alkaline water regularly. Also, I went on intermittent fasting and vegan diets. All these actions got me this far then why would I think any different now. I haven't seen or talked to a doctor in over eight years. My weight may have been a little high at 290 pounds; however I "carried" it well. As a truck driver, my diet wasn't the greatest but as I stated I tried to balance it out.

Now as a truck driver you are affected about what goes on with the economy pretty quickly. And that is what started to occur. I worked for a placement company that places drivers on a day to day basis. Sometimes you would get lucky and find an assignment that lasts for months. That was my assignment until covid caused Georgia to shut down. Now the need for placement drivers was going thin unless you wanted to go over the road and travel. I been there and done that and was tired of sleeping in the trucks and bad food.

Needless to say, they didn't need me to come back. That led to intermittent assignments and a broken sleep cycle. Consequently, my pay was reduced and the stress was building up inside. With stress comes comfort meals, which usually means carbs, fat, and fast food. My diet of alkaline water and fasting was out the window. Since my work schedule was looking bleak I decided to take a short trip out of town to clear my head.

After a couple of days out of town, I started heading back to help my child's mother, Constance move. On my way back I was tired and needed sleep. I stopped a few times to get some rest. It was unusual because I was a truck driver and should have been able to drive back. I took it as nothing big. Once I arrived at the house, I took another nap.

A muffled "Wake up" was all I heard as I looked over at the driver's side window. Constance was standing there. I rolled the window down and opened up an energy drink. "Oh, you ready now?" as I took a sip.

"Yes I am," she replied. I took another sip, and started my van, and unlocked the doors. We were headed to the U-Haul store off of Fulton Industrial Boulevard. She got the truck and I drove it back to the house, loaded it then went to the apartment. So far so good, I was feeling a little tired but it was understandable, knowing how far I drove the night before.

The truck was almost unloaded when I took a break. I sat at the end of the tailgate to get myself together. I guess the moving and steps and heat were getting to me. She saw how I was looking and asked if we should get some help. I initially refused. Then as I got up and felt a little light-headed, I agreed. Once I agreed, I knew something was not exactly right. I have been through many is situations where I pushed through the physical and mental pain to accomplish the goal ahead. But this was different somehow, someway.

We picked up some help and reloaded the truck and got to the apartment. This time I didn't get out the truck once I parked it. I tilted my head back and slouched down, closed my eyes, and was knocked out. I woke up to my son, Lynden, asking me if I wanted something to eat. I said yes and a bottle of water. After the food and water, I went back to sleep.

The truck got unloaded and we dropped off the guys. Little did I know my health was deteriorating and I had no clue about what was about to occur.

CHAPTER TWO

A Blast from the Past

There have been times where I had to accomplish a set planned workout goal for myself. And that goal was set and could not be overridden or failed. Usually, these goals are for working out or fitness. An example would be when I told myself I must walk up Stone Mountain two times with a twenty-pound vest on in the middle of the summer. Now this goal was to take place in the morning. However, if you know anything about Georgia summers the morning is still humid. So after my first walk up and back down I was feeling a little winded. The sweat was pouring and the muscles started to ache if I stood still. Luckily I didn't stand still long.

After the second up and down the mountain, I knew it was a wrap. I was drenched with sweat and the ache was turning against me. The walk to the car was baby steps at the most. After taking the wet clothes off and drinking water and a sports drink, I was coming back to life enough to drive home. Now, this event was pretty bad but nothing like the next two situations.

I called this one; chocolate doesn't melt on the sidewalk or the Savannah incident. A year or more ago, I left Atlanta to go to Savannah for a change of scenery and pace. I needed something different and Savannah was right around the corner and near the ocean, without being too far from Atlanta. During my stay there I was driving trucks and stayed in a weekly room. During work, I listened to motivational people with different mindsets. That's when I clicked on David Goggins, a former Navy SEAL. Listening to him talk and the things that he had been through motivated me to get his audiobook. And that's when it clicked in me to do more physically to see how far I could push myself.

So, there was this park about two miles from where I was staying. I mapped out the route and saw that it was about six miles or so if I walked to the park and walked around it then headed back. Six miles that was a walk in the park, no pun intended. I got up one morning drank a lot of water and filled my camel pack with water. A camel pack is a book bag with a plastic-type water jug inside, you can fill with water. And a tube comes out of the top goes through the book bag so you can drink without stopping. Imagine a hospital IV bag with a tube in it for drinking.

Once I was hydrated and my bag was full of water I grabbed my headphones and headed out. The morning was the usual muggy humid weather with no rain. I had motivational music and speeches playing in my ear the whole time. I made it back to my room feeling a little taxing but it wasn't like walking Stone Mountain. Mission accomplished now time for a shower, relax, and get ready for the next day. Yes, I was getting ready to do the same thing the next day.

Two days six miles that shouldn't be hard. That's what I was telling myself when I initially planned the route. What I didn't plan for was the way my body was responding to the first six miles.

Before walking that first six miles, I hadn't worked out or walked that distance for a few months. My mind was focused on accomplishing the goal while my brain and body was recovering from the "walk to the park."

The next day I was not feeling any muscle soreness or any side effects from the previous day's walk. I drank water and waited for my urine to be clear before I headed back out. I followed the same procedure as the day before, I drank water then pour some in my camel pack, grabbed my headphones, and started walking.

Now getting to the park was easy. As I got halfway around I hit what runners call "the wall." It's a feeling that no matter what you do you can't go faster. I found myself sitting down for the first time on a park bench, going through my protocols to assess what was going on with me. The only answer I could come up with was, I need to push harder. So that's what I did, I pushed on, only to get to the next park bench. I went through my protocols and realized something was not going well inside of me. I was feeling lightheaded and pouring in sweat but it wasn't that hot out. I knew then I needed to get back to the room.

I walked as fast as I could which wasn't fast at all. I got out of the park and made it to a corner gas station. I bought some water and a sports drink, slowly drank them while sitting on the curb. At this point, I was exhausted and still sweating. I sat down and started going in and out of consciousness. I could feel the air conditioning from the front door as people were going in and out. One customer saw me laying there and brought me a bottle of water. I mustered up enough strength to thank him as he handed it to me.

The water was a lifesaver as I drifted back to sleep. Then my inner voice spoke to me and as clear as day I heard, "Carter if you don't get up now, you will never get up." Needless to say, I jumped up like a jack in the box, still tired and groggy I walked over to a cement pole, laid my hands on the top, and rested my head on my hands.

I stood there which seem like hours, still tired, sweating, and groggy. I told myself I got to keep moving to get back to my room. Now from the gas station to my room had to be about a mile. It took me an hour and a half to get there. I struggled to get the key in the lock. But once I got to my room I was done. There was a gallon of water there that I sipped on for hours whenever I woke up enough to sip. I laid down with my arms and legs extended to prevent cramping. Something I learned years before from the Peachtree road race incident.

The Peachtree road race incident was my previous incident which included a near-total body failure. The race itself was not the issue; it was the total lack of planning. Before the road race, I was jogging around Stone Mountain about twice a week. Stone Mountain was approximately five miles and the road race was a little over six miles. What's an extra mile, right?

On the day of the race, I drank Gatorade and had water the staples of a pre-race hydration. And as usual, the weather was a factor. The fourth of July is always humid. Even though the race started early in the morning, it was still high humidity. As the race started everything was great. A slow, steady jog at first. I was jogging the race with Evans, my academy classmate. We finished the race and then turned around and walked back to the starting line. That's where I parked the car.

Our walk back was becoming an adventure in itself. We were getting dehydrated and tired as the sun was relentless. We made it back to the car and I drove towards the house. I say towards the house because I didn't make it there. On the way there, I was slowly getting drowsy and tired. I pulled into the QT and woke him up before I passed out.

I don't remember exactly how I got into my house but the assumption is Evans help me get in there. Once I got inside I laid on the floor and drank some water. I sat up to lean on the couch with my legs bent, wrong idea. The cramps came through like lightning bolts in both my legs. As I tried to straighten them all I could think about was someone pulling apart a crab leg to get the meat out. Several moments passed as I continued to straighten my legs. Eventually, I accomplish the task. My legs were now straight but now my arms wanted some attention. I immediately straighten them out. Now I'm leaned up against my couch on the floor looking like a starfish. I waited for the pain in my arms to subside so I could drink some more water. After another sip, it was sleepy time. I repeated this process until I was able to move without cramping. Oh, what a day I was having, but I survived so I'm better for it.

CHAPTER THREE
All Hell broke Loose

From the day after I helped Constance move to the day I went to a hotel was a blur to me. During this time Covid had its grip on me. I was in and out of consciousness. I was told that I had a bowel movement while I was sleeping in my son's bed. I was also on a nebulizer and albuterol to help with my breathing. I wasn't eating. One of the few moments I do remember is holding Constance hand and telling her that I never felt this way before and then I passed out.

One of my moments of clarity came as Constance woke me up and told me, either you go to the hospital or you go to a hotel, but you are not going to die here. Well, that was clear. I chose the hotel. She took me to a hotel and I got up the strength to walk inside and get to my room. After checking up on me she left. I was actually doing fine. Or maybe it was the moving that got the blood and fluids flowing that gave me false hope.

Mentally I was doing fine. I have been through these dark times, Peachtree, Savannah, before, and this was just another one of those times. I knew I was going to be alright because my body knew the drill. Little did I know this wasn't a drill, it was a full-on fire.

At this point, I'm losing the battle with covid. So I'm in the hotel on April 06 and much of that time there was a blur too. I don't remember going to the room or unpacking my suitcase. For the most part, this book from here until I get out of ICU is from the perspective of my mother and Constance.

After I was dropped off and secure in the hotel room Constance called my mother and gave her my hotel room key. On April 07 my mom checked up on me and I was groggy but ok. I pushed myself to make her feel better. Later that day my mother left me and went home. The next day April 08, she came back. When she got into the room she could see I had labored breathing. She called Constance and was told to call the front desk to have 911 called. Because calling from the room could confuse the 911 dispatch side. My mother called the front desk and the fire department showed up. I was then transported to the nearest hospital. In the meantime, my mother was frantic while trying to get my belongings from the hotel room. The hotel would not let her back in the room. At this time covid was being treated as a very contagious problem and the room was blocked off as was part of the hotel.

Needless to say, she got what she could and headed to the hospital. At the hospital, she was told, if I made it the next 24 hours I was lucky. Wow, imagine hearing that as they take your only son away on a stretcher and not allowing you to see him. The feelings and emotions were on an epic scale.

The hospital could not allow my mother to see me or tell her what was going on. There was a nurse or two who would contact her to let her know that I was still alive. My mother made it a point to stay in touch and ask many questions about me. One question, in particular, was about my "output." In regular terms, my output was urine or feces. Once she found out my output of urine was low, she told the nurses, "that's not my son, he urines a lot." What I found out later is that I had a condom catheter over my penis. Long story short, men have difficulty urinating when the penis tip is squeezed. The condom catheter was removed and an inserted catheter was used and the urine flowed like the mighty Mississippi. Interestingly enough I remember that part. Well, at least the part where my penis was hurting from the catheter. That was one of the few times that I woke up from the drug-induced coma. Yes, a drug-induced coma. I'll explain why later.

Now I'm in the hospital and my mother is worried, rightfully so and the news gets back to my son. Initially, he was alright with it. He knew his father was the type of man who would do workouts in the rain, walk in the cold, and push himself. My son showed a strong front when the news came to him. Then after a few days, the news hit him. As I stated before these are not my words but the words of the people involved.

He told me, at first he was ok because he knows his father. But during the next few days, he felt differently. He cried and cried but didn't want to wake up his mother. He got into the bathtub crying, texting but it was late night and no one was responding except one friend, Kenya. Kenya was friends with Constance going on decades. She was the voice that my son listened to, to get some type of grounding on this situation. Side note, I greatly appreciate that. My son talked to Kenya and calm down. Later that morning when Constance woke up, she looked at her phone and saw all the messages from people concerned about Lynden, which then made her concerned. However, by then my son was sleep.

CHAPTER FOUR
Miracle Patient

When I say a miracle patient I'm not talking as if I am some type of superman. I am taking this from the doctors and nurses who worked on me when I arrived at the hospital. One male nurse, in particular, was working that night and seen me come in looking pale and barely breathing. I had a blood oxygen level at around 45 percent. Just know that the level of a normal breathing person is 90 percent or better. I should have already been dead and gone. So when they told my mother that I had a fifty-fifty chance, they were not lying.

Now, this is where Covid is different than the common cold or flu virus. Covid looks and seeks out the cracks in your health. Almost, like software that looks for vulnerable places on your computer. So while I'm in the hospital under a drug-induced coma, covid was going to work. Covid located many of my cracks and started a process of making them bigger. The first crack was my lungs.

As I stated earlier my blood oxygen level was around 45 percent. My lungs were literally closing on me, preventing my blood from getting oxygen and getting rid of carbon dioxide. I was slowly choking to death. While this was occurring my heart was trying to pump more blood to get the oxygen level up. This caused a mild heart attack to occur. Once I got on the ventilator and got somewhat stabilized other tests where conducted. There was an ulcer found along with liver issues.

The longer I stayed in the coma on the ventilator, my kidneys stopped working. Now with this list of problems and issues, covid wasn't done yet. But let's recap before we move on. There are my lungs and breathing issues. My heart is now beating at less than 10 percent. The ulcer is possibly causing bowel issues. And we can't forget about the kidneys, which both of them have stopped working.

One thing among most covid sufferers is blood clots. Blood clots seem to be the calling card for covid and I had them in my right leg. So during one of my few conscious moments in the ICU, I was advised on the clots. The doctors recommended a strainer put in my leg to prevent the clot from coming loose and causing other issues. I agreed and the strainer was placed in my right leg.

Also, during my ICU stay while I was comatose there was a decision made to provide me with Covid antibodies. My mother was contacted and arrived at the hospital to give the signature needed. Once that was done, the antibodies were administered and the waiting game continued.

Days later I'm still alive and on the ventilator. The male nurse who seen me come in was surprised I was still alive. He called my mother to tell her how I was doing better. My mother appreciated the call and thanked him for the updates and help he assisted her with.

CHAPTER FIVE

Now What?

Now it's twenty or so days in the ICU, I'm waking up more and noticing my surroundings. One of the things that got my attention was my hands were tied to the bed rails. I don't know about you but I don't think that is a usual thing to see when you are in a hospital ICU. So, I was wondering, why am I tied up? Along with being tied up, I had weighted boots velcroed to my feet. I later found out the weights were for blood circulation and prevention of certain bed sores on your feet. Ok, I understood that, but why were my hands tied to the bed?

I'll just say I had a few "elevated" episodes while I was in ICU. And by elevated episodes I mean highly raised blood pressure as I was trying to take out the ventilator and other things attached to me. I don't remember these episodes or the outcomes but

I'm still here so everything must have worked out. During the earlier episodes, a decision had to be made to keep me sleep as long as possible to prevent more of them. And the sleep drug of choice used on me was Propofol. For the people who are not familiar with Propofol, it's the drug that killed Michael Jackson. The drug's street name is "milk of amnesia." Well, that explains why my memory was not so good. With this information, it was interesting to see that Propofol was used over eighty times during my stay. When I say used, I'm saying it was listed over 80 times on my medical bill. I'm not a doctor but if it's listed that many times it had to be used at least half if not more.

During those long periods of sleep, people asked me if I had dreams. I can't tell you about the dreams because I don't remember having any. The only thing I clearly remember is having out of body experiences. I was floating above my physical body. The room was different less like a hospital room more like a hotel room. I could see myself and there was a sense of peace and quietness. I didn't float away or feel any pain. Just a peacefulness that's like nothing I knew before. I read about astral projection where people could leave their physical bodies and go to other places. But that was not the thinking I was having during these times. I can't tell you how long they lasted. However, I can tell you they were real.

Now that I am waking up more often and recovering well, doctors are talking to me. This goes back to the miracle patient. There wasn't a doctor or anyone who worked on me that didn't tell me, they can't believe I made it through. Some of them would look bug-eyed to see me awake and moving a little. I still had the ventilator attached along with the heart monitor and of course IV tubes. When I was fully awake and aware I can see why they had to put me to sleep. Seeing all those tubes and wires, who wouldn't be a little freaked out? After a few more days the day of reckoning came, I was getting the ventilator out. Oh boy, I couldn't wait. Taking it out and breathing on my own was a good day for me. Now I just had to have an oxygen tube on my nose. I'll take that over a ventilator any day. The ventilator is gone, I'm speaking better, hands are untied, it was time to move out of ICU

CHAPTER SIX

The Aftermath

Now that I'm upstairs out of ICU I should be going home soon, wrong. This is the time where I learn all the things Covid did to me and the effects. I knew I had tubes hooked up to me to feed and give me water but the fact that I haven't eaten anything was messing with my mind. So days rolled by and I'm working with a speech therapist and she is slowly giving me crackers and pieces of cubed peaches. All of this is because when the ventilator is in your throat and it can cause issues. Primarily swallowing issues where food may somehow get into your lungs instead of your stomach. So precautions are taken so that doesn't happen, peaches and crackers.

This also goes for water. the only water I could have is from the sip of this sponge they called the "turtle." It was more or less a popsicle stick with a green sponge on the end. So they would soak it in water and give it to me. Even at this point, I was still having issues swallowing. But man o man that water was good.

Talking was also an issue at the beginning. I just knew I was going to go right back to the way I was before covid, nope. I was struggling to say words and definitely long sentences. This was a trying time for me and the nurses or others coming into my room. At times it seems as if I was a burden to some of them. The feeling of helplessness was seeping in. Understand I had been through some trying times in my health as I wrote earlier, so this was huge for me. However, I stayed focused and kept telling myself, this will be over soon and it was.

As the days rolled by I got better at talking and moving around. I wasn't walking yet, just moving around in bed. The speech therapist was satisfied with my progress and I was able to eat more solid foods. Now I know I don't have to mention this but hospital food isn't the greatest. So when I was able to get access to my cell phone I called people on "the outside" to get me some real food. Then when my first "outside" meal came, it was chicken wings. That's when I noticed my taste buds were no good. All this time I thought it was the hospital food. Then another meal I requested came, Chick-fil-A, the same outcome. It's interesting to see and eat food you can't taste or smell. It's almost like a magic trick someone is playing on you. So I'm thinking ok let me request something I know will work, lemonade. This had to work, I love lemonade. The tart taste will wake up my taste buds and I'll be good to go. Nope, my master plan did not work. I was feeling anxious now.

More days rolled by almost like the movie, Groundhog Day, where every day seemed like the same day. Breakfast was usually two sausages, toast with some type of eggs, and grits. Then the nurse comes in with medicine for me. Breaking that monotony up was the phlebotomist who took my blood. At one point I swear I was getting blood taken every four to six hours. One time I asked why the blood was being taken so many times? The answer was, the different medicines were being tested and the doctors needed to get the dosages right. That made sense to me, even if it didn't that wasn't going to stop them from getting the blood.

Then a huge change up occurred, which would turn my life around. I was getting sent to dialysis. Three days a week Monday, Wednesday, Friday. That was almost too much to handle. I understood the other parts of my body that had failed but was recovering. But knowing the kidneys were not coming back online was a blow. Dialysis took about three hours from beginning to end. And on one occasion the blood clots, clogged up the machine and it had to be stopped. Imagine seeing and hearing that news. The only good thing that was good coming out of dialysis was the way it put me to sleep. The procedure itself wasn't bad. It's the recovery that takes your energy.

Around this time a decision was made by my kidney doctor to insert a port to make dialysis easier. For the past week or so the dialysis machine was connected to the ports on my right arm. Since those ports were eventually going to be removed, a more permanent port needed to be added. Imagine my surprise when I heard this. The surgery was pretty quick. They inserted a tube in my neck connecting to the main artery with the ports stitched to my chest. A clear plastic film was placed over the stitching so they would not become infected. From time to time the stitching bled a little and the clear plastic film had to be changed out.

The ports were cool for a couple of days until out of nowhere the place where the tube was connected to my neck started to bleed. This would have not been an issue if it wasn't for the massive amount of blood thinners I was on. So now instead of a normal bleeding situation, there was a good flow coming out. I contacted the nurse several times before one came in and addressed the issue. By that time my bed looked like a crime scene. Later it was found out I bleed enough to need a blood transfusion. I did receive some plasma to replace the plasma I lost and luckily the tube in my neck never bleed again.

Some people would tell you they got to rest while in the hospital, well that wasn't my case. Feeling hot sometimes cold, machines beeping and of course, visits from different people to check your progress. Then there are the lab people pulling blood. Don't get me wrong I am thankful for being alive and getting better, however, if you had a long stay anywhere you know what I mean. I fully understand why some people just don't make it. The anxiety, depression, lack of sleep, and just simply not knowing when you will be released can take its toll.

Then one day the good news starts coming in. I wake up as usual and get wheeled into dialysis. I get comfortable, turn the TV on, and get ready for the three-hour procedure. As I'm watching a commercial the curtain is pulled back and the technician tells me

I'm done. I smile and ask, what happened? She tells me the kidney doctor called and stated my kidneys have come back online and are functioning enough to stop dialysis. If that wasn't the best news I heard in a while. My blood pressure went up a little in excitement. Later that day the kidney doctor came to my room and explained the blood test to me and how pleased he was at my progress. However, there were ports in my chest to facilitate the dialysis procedure. He was not going to go as far as removing the ports until he sees a definitive blood test of my kidney function. And of course, I wasn't happy with that but it made sense.

The good news kept pouring in after that. Another technician came in a day later to test my blood oxygen level to see if I will need a tank after I get discharged. I told her honestly that I have been removing the oxygen tube periodically just because it felt uncomfortable. Well, I guess my body adapted because my oxygen levels were ninety-eight percent consistent. So no oxygen was needed. My eating was getting better. I got removed from the special diet to regular food. And my walking was stable enough and improving to get signed off on that too.

At this point I'm feeling like I'm on top of the world, so when am I going home? That answer would seem to be an elusive one. The answer I was given was, there still need to be some other blood tests, and to ensure a rise in my white blood count was not going to be an issue. All I could hear is a balloon popping. I wasn't too discouraged, I got this far and "it will be over soon". A day or two later a doctor came into my room midday. I never saw him before. He was telling me of the results from tests and he was sending me home today. I was shocked, so I asked him, like today, today? He looked at me and said, yes, after he finishes his paperwork on me I'm going home. He looked at me and said, you're ok with that? I said hell yeah.

I called my mother and told her. She said they were going to release me tomorrow. I told her what that doctor said and she wasn't sure what was going on. So she called the nurse who was in contact with her about my release. Moments later that nurse came into my room and told me my mother called and said I was being released today. I told her yes ma'am, the doctor said as soon as he is done with the paperwork. The nurse even looked shocked and left the room. She came back later and said I guess you are going home today. I packed up some personal belongings and waited for the wheelchair to head out.

CHAPTER SEVEN

Home Sweet, Home?

Before I head home I need to add a little backstory. Before getting Covid I was a regional truck driver. I didn't have an apartment because it would not have been reasonable or economical. So the plan was to get a room in an extended stay for a month. Everything sounded good until the plan had to be executed. Knowing how much a room for a month was, I questioned who was paying and so forth. The answers came out was, don't worry about it, it will get done. Since I'm a planning person that worried me. Not that I didn't want things to go well, but this wasn't looking good for the home team. But now the moment of truth was upon us.

I was released and headed to an extended stay. This particular extended stay was not part of the plan, it was a last-minute hail mary. I couldn't worry about that right now; I was just happy to be out of the hospital. I thanked everyone involved and relaxed. The days passed by and the question of another extended stay was coming up. At this point, I was getting some money from disability and family. I used it to pay for another room for a week.

Now I'm feeling some type of way about how the promises were broken. When I was told to don't worry about it raised a red flag. At one point I was told to think positive and pray. There is only so much positivity and prayer that is going to come out of this situation. This is more of a plan that was not properly executed. Needless to say, I made things work out with the help of Constance.

I appreciate the concern and care that my family showed me while I was in the hospital. I just wish there was a better plan in place. Having to deal with this living situation and trying to recover was too much. I learned a lot and am still learning.

I am still regaining my strength back and some of my weight. My taste buds haven't fully recovered but I know they are. My heart and lungs and other organs are getting better, especially my kidneys. I still have issues walking as my right leg seems to not be as strong as my left. My right leg was where the strainer was put in for the blood clots. SSI disability also feels like I'm better as they cut me off the program. The letter in so many words read, you are good enough to get some job, now get it. Thank you, SSI. I still have more appointments to go to. The post monitoring process probably will never end. As more is found out about Covid more questions arise.

Now here comes the unknown parts and mystery of covid. Yes, I can get covid again. There is no guarantee that it will be less severe or just minor symptoms. Will there be a vaccine? And if there is, will it work against Covid for people who already had it? Because, like the flu shot which contains inactive flu viruses, will this cause a negative reaction in prior Covid patients. There are also long term Covid sufferers that will need additional care. The medical community is still learning about how Covid is affecting people, so there are no real concrete answers. And not having answers doesn't give people peace of mind. Covid is here to stay. The effects of covid are numerous and some are still being figured out. The hope is there will be a better understanding and better treatment.

CHAPTER EIGHT
Final Thoughts

First and foremost covid is real. Why there is a debate about this is beyond me. The thinking that some people have that "only" a few hundred thousand died of covid doesn't mean that it is dangerous. That type of thinking is dangerous. I have to admit I was a little skeptical of covid myself. Now that I have first-hand experience, I'm a believer. However, I do not want someone to have to go through my experience just to prove a point. That is one of the main reasons why I wrote this book was to put a human face on Covid.

As my body recovers slowly but surely the stress of being in the hospital is over. The doctors telling me my body was recovering well and the internal organs that were failing or had issues were good. Now there is one part of my body that I was concerned about recovering to its full pre-covid condition, my manhood. There has been only one other time where I was concerned about it and that was in basic military training. While in training we were told it was normal for us to experience a change in function because of the stress training puts on the mind. As for this hospital stress I understood why the function had changed. Once I left the hospital and got relaxed, the functioning went back to normal, even with the different medications.

While I reflect on my ordeal I am grateful. But as they say, the hard part is the recovery. Since I am used to going all out and working out to my fullest, this new phase is something to get used to, and it's hard. I am still in pain when I walk. I can't lift simple heavy grocery bags up a flight of stairs. The knee and elbow joint pains are still there. I know time will heal me. I also know I won't be the person I was before Covid, so I'll take it one day at a time.

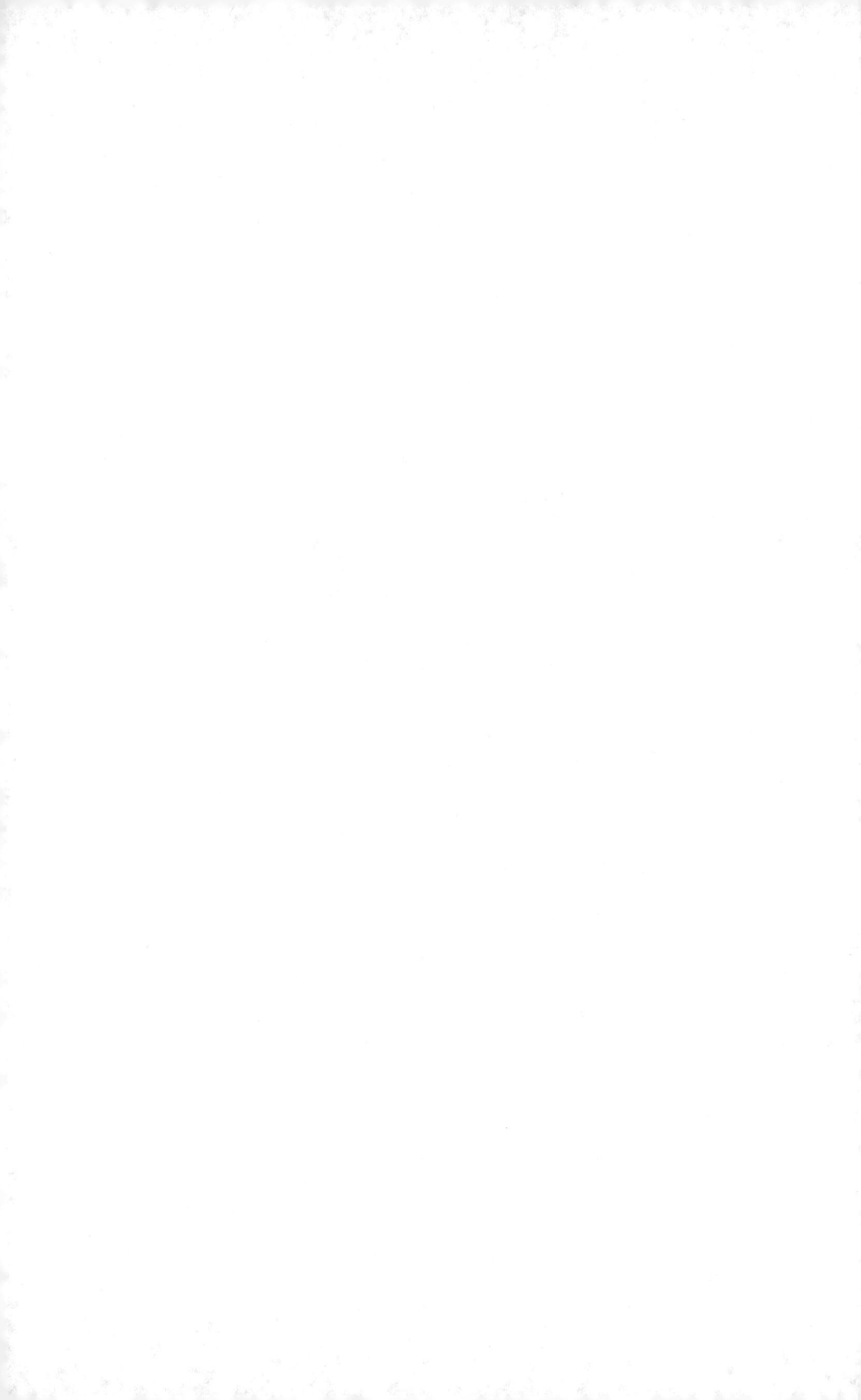